Chronicles of an Autistic Child

Part One:

The Childs View

Prologue

Hello, my name is Ricky, and this is my story. It started on a cold December morning in 2006 at a little after nine in the morning. This is the day that I was born by cesarean section, and I weighed over eight pounds and was twenty inches long. Everything started out so normal.

I was my mommies first little boy and her second child. However, what my mom didn't know is that through the coming years I would be throwing a lot of curb balls at her. You see I was not a typical child from the very beginning, but no one could have predicted just how different things were going to be with me.

I was never a crier as a baby. I loved just laying in my crib and listening to my favorite movie, "Cars" with Lightening McQueen. I was an easy-going baby for the first few years. Though I did not develop the normal skills right off my mom was not yet worried. I mean every child grows differently right?

I was not walking or talking, but I was rolling around a lot and bumping into things. I didn't really like being held so I spent a lot of time playing on a blanket on the floor when I wasn't in my crib. I enjoyed just being mostly on my own.

My first few months as a baby were the easiest for my mom, because I was easier to please than I am now. In the beginning my mom did not know that there was something different about me. She didn't know that in a few years she would have her whole world flipped upside down, because of me. No one really knew then just how different I am.

But the journey was just beginning for my family. It really was just beginning for me too. My case however is different from others that my mom has studied or even read about or seen. I am an autistic child, but I am not your typical autistic child. Through these chronicles I will explain just how different I really am and share my experiences.

Then my parents and sisters will share their thoughts and beliefs as well, so as to provide the view from more than just my own side. I hope that by sharing this it will help others to understand what children like me go through on a day to day basis. Also, I hope it will help others to understand that this is not easy and for some may not get any easier, while for others it may.

Chapter 1

The first thing my mom was told about me was when I was three months old and diagnosed with asthma. I was put on breathing treatments. I hated those because I had to wear a mask and it felt weird.

Don't get me wrong my mom is a strong lady, she has faced most of the problems with me all by herself. I admire my mom a lot for the courage that she has always shown. That was really the only thing that happened in my first few months. It wasn't until I was a year old that my mom started noticing that I was different.

When I reached my first birthday and had not yet learned or even attempted to learn to walk or talk, that is when my mom became worried. She began then to suspect that I was not a normal baby, and she was right. I was not even babbling like most babies do when they are young and trying to get the understanding of using their lungs and mouths.

You see for my mom it was difficult to understand why I was not walking or talking. I mean my older sister started talking at six months old and was walking at around the same age. Why was I so different? Was I meant to challenge my mom?

I did not know and neither did she. Finally, at eighteen months old I began to try my feet out and take my first steps. At twenty-two months, I was diagnosed with my first diagnoses, it was called Pervasive Development Disorder Not Otherwise Specified (PDD-NOS). Do you know what that is? I'll explain, PDD-NOS is a mild way of saying that a child is not developing correctly or at the pace that the people around them believes that they should, but yet they also do not know why that child is not developing normally.

However, that diagnoses was changed when I reached thirty-three months of age. I was then diagnosed with High-Functioning Autism (HFA). The doctors told my mom that I had to have therapy to learn a different way to communicate so that I could talk to her. So, mom signed me up for a program called Babies Can't Wait.

The therapist came to visit with me at home, so that I would be more comfortable. She began to teach me about my body parts, by singing a song with me every time she came. She also taught me and my mom how to use a few ASL (American Sign

Language) signs to help us be able to communicate. I thought that was pretty cool.

With this new knowledge of being able to talk with my hands, it then made it easier for me to communicate with my mom. I was able to tell her what I needed, and she was able to understand me. It was amazing finally being able to tell my mom things even if it was just with my hands.

This is how my second year of life proceeded. I'd sign something with my hands and my mom would understand me and help however she was able too.

Chapter 2

A couple months before I was to turn three years old the therapist stopped coming to the house and mom said I was going to school. All I could think when she said that was I'm to young for school. However, I was changed from the Babies Can't Wait program over to the local school just before I turned three years old. Turned out it was a special school.

It was a school especially for the kids that were special in many different ways. I attended the special needs school for almost two whole years. In the middle of my second year at the preschool for special kids, I finally discovered my voice.

I began to talk a bit. Not really understandable words, but words none the less. I was saying things like wawa (translation- Dada), and baba (translation- bottle). I did not know at the time how to say the actual words, but that didn't matter because my family understood either way. That was all that really mattered at that time.

Throughout my years at the special needs school I discovered who I was. I discovered my feet a bit better than I had been doing and even though I was walking mostly on my tiptoes my mom said she was just happy to see me walking better. I was no longer stumbling over my own feet. However, these were also the beginning of my trouble years. I got in trouble the first time in school when I was 3 years old for throwing crayons at my classmates. I was just talked to about how it was impolite to throw things.

I didn't really listen to that though because I got in trouble again when I was 4 years old for throwing matchbox cars at my teacher. I was punished with a timeout at school for doing that. That was my first punishment ever really. First couple of years were rocky, but my mom made it work.

My mom was dating a guy who became her second husband for all of 4 months when I first received my diagnoses. This guy did not help my mom with me at all, honestly for my first 8 years after my original diagnoses no one really helped my mom. She pretty much had to raise me by herself for my first 8 years. The past 3 years however have been easier on her.

Her new husband has been a huge support system for my mom and what she goes through with me on a daily basis. Though this is totally off subject so back to the story.

I finally entered normal Pre-Kindergarten at the age of 5. By then I was talking a little more clearly. My words were sometimes hard to understand, but after 4 years of silence my mom was just happy to hear me talking.

I learned a lot during my pre-kindergarten year, but none the less my words for the most part still seemed to escape me.

Chapter 3

My first few years in regular school was spent discovering who I was and how to do certain things. My kindergarten year I do not remember much of, but my first-grade year was the first time that I ever really got into serious trouble at school. That was the first year the teachers actually called my mom over something that I had done.

That was the first and only time that my mom let the principal at school paddle me. I had gotten into trouble with my teacher and decided that I did not want to listen to her. She called the principal and he came to get me. He picked me up and was going to tote me out of the classroom so that he could talk to me.

However, he made the mistake of setting me on the floor just outside of the classroom. So, I kicked him and took off back into the classroom. I decided I was going to hide under the table and not come out. That is when the teacher made the decision to call my mom.

My mom was not happy about having to make a trip to the school. I could tell when she came to the door of the classroom that she was not happy with me or with how I was acting. You see up until this point I had not made my mom as upset as she was when she had to come to the school. The teacher explained to my mom that I was refusing to come out from under the table.

So, my mom sat on the floor and talked to me and slowly coaxed me out from under the table. I crawled out and sat in my mom's lap, because I thought that I was not going to get into trouble. Though it turned out that I thought wrong, because I did get into trouble. That was the day that my mom talked to the principal and he suggested that she should let him paddle me.

My mom thought about it for a whole day before giving the principal permission to paddle me. I did not cry though when I was paddled. I looked at the principal and told him that it didn't hurt at all. I know it was not a smart thing to say, but I did not think about it at that time. I just said the first thing that popped into my head.

Chapter 4

My second-grade year we moved back to Forsyth and I was attending school with my two sisters. That was my next eventful year. I got in trouble that year for stealing trying to steal Lego blocks from the school. That was also the year that I ended up with a sprained arm. Another kid pulled me off the jungle gym at school and I got hurt.

What had my mom most upset though was when I got into trouble for trying to steal. My mom was not happy with me at all for that. Though I did not take heed to the fact that I should not do it and kept trying to steal. I even tried stealing things from stores in town.

My mom caught me and took me to the police station because she said that was not how she had raised me and that was not something I was going to do. The officer talked to me about the consequences of my actions and even showed me the juvenile holding cell. Then he told my mom that he felt the best course of action was for me to write letters to all the places I had tried to steal from and to my sisters and mom apologizing for my actions.

My mom agreed, and the officer said I was to bring the notes to him after they were done, and he would deliver them to where they belonged. So, that was what my mom had me do. Seeing the Juvenile holding call scared me.

My third-grade year my family moved out of state to Virginia and I went to school there. It was an uneventful year. I barely got in any trouble at all other than an occasional reprimand for talking during class. I had no major trouble that year. I did make a lot of friends that year though.

That was also the year my mom met and married our step-dad. He is awesome. Even though sometimes I feel that he is being stricter with me than he is with my sisters. I know that he only does it because he is doing what he thinks is best for me. I respect that about him, even if I do not always show him.

My fourth-grade year I was good all year long and then decide to get into trouble close to the end of the year. I once again was in trouble for trying to steal. My teacher had caught me trying to steal from the school book fair. I broke my principals' heart when I got caught. She had been so proud of me up until that point and I let her and my mom and dad down.

I ended up receiving my first ever ISS (In School Suspension) that year and my mom was not a happy camper when that happened. She took away my video games and my tv and said it would be a long while before I got them back. I didn't blame her though, I knew what I had done was wrong and yet I had still done it.

I was also made to write letters to my teacher, my principal and the librarian apologizing for what I had done. My mom took me to school herself on the day I was to deliver them and walked with me to hand to deliver them to each person. I was so embarrassed, but I knew I deserved the punishment that I was getting.

You see I may be diagnosed with High-functioning Autism, ADHD (Attention Deficit Hyperactivity Disorder), ODD (Oppositional Defiant Disorder) and child Bipolar Disorder, but those things are not what defines me. Those things do not control me.

I am what I myself choose to make myself. Even with everything that I am diagnosed with I know the difference between right and wrong. I know when I have done somethings that I shouldn't have done. That does not stop me from doing it, but I know when I am wrong, at least most of the time.

I got into the band my fourth-grade year. Tested into it with the highest score in my school. I was proud of my accomplishment and enjoyed playing my instrument. I also made the Lego League that year. If only I had not gotten in trouble, then my year would have been awesome all the way through.

Chapter 5

My fifth-grade year I was still in band but decided to drop it after a couple of months. It was a good year though. My mom moved us once again, but this time we moved to South Georgia and got us a lot closer to the beach. I like our new school. I was really good my fifth-grade year.

This year I am a sixth-grader and I have rejoined the band. I even tried out and made the football team, but I ended up dropping it. I did not like the idea of our team being cussed at by our assistant coach. This year has been an okay year. There are somethings that I could do differently, but I guess it's a little late for that.

I got my second ever ISS this year for hitting another boy who had been on my football team. Then my third one for farting in class during an active shooter lockdown of the school. Both things that probably could have and should have been avoided, but I ignored what I knew was right and did what I wanted to do.

I have learned many things throughout my eleven years. This year I will be twelve on my birthday and my moms' hope with sharing my story of my years up to now is that hopefully my story will help other kids or even other parents to understand what it is like to be a child living with Autism.

I hope that my story will be an inspiration of sorts to other kids like me who are living on the Autism Spectrum. No, I do not hope that these kids will try to mimic the bad things that I have done, but instead to learn from them and know that they are not the correct things to have been done.

I want them to understand that even though I was diagnosed with all of these mental problems that I am what controls my actions, just as they are what controls their actions.

Chapter 6

You see I have struggled constantly to get to where I am today. I am a child who is completely different from any other. I am different from most of my peers. No one can really understand what it is like to be an eleven-year-old boy living with Autism. No one can really understand the constant struggle that I have daily with myself just to do the right thing and stay out of trouble.

You see everyone I meet looks at me as if I am different or strange. I show out in public, even when I really have what appears to be no real reason too. My mom has tried her hardest though out the years to help the people around me understand that I am different. Though most of them just tell her that she is babying me and that she needs to stop.

My friends, and cousins, do not want to play with me and most of the time my sisters only want to fight with me. My family thinks that I am emotional and out of control and most of them have told my mom that they believe the best thing for me would be for her to send me away. My mom on the other hand does not believe this to be true.

My formal name is Ricky. I am an 11-year-old boy living with Autism. I am ranked on the ASD scale. But I am not Autism. That is not what defines me as a person. I am a child unlike any other. I have melt downs and show out. I get upset if things do not always go just the way that I want them too.

I am hyperactive and sometimes have a hard time staying focused on what I should be doing. When I was younger, I was diagnosed Significant Developmental Delays and Speech problems. I have now out grown most of that. I talk pretty clearly now. I am still super hyper though all the time. I have a hard time sitting still a lot of the time.

But I am a child, no matter what all the doctors say about me I am still just a child. I am an extra special child, who loves cars, trucks, trains, and planes. Anything really that has wheels on it. I am a child who shows out and needs medication to help me to control myself. I am a child, an extra special child who is loved by his mommy, daddy, and sisters. I am extra special.

God made me special for a reason and later I will make something great of myself. Doctors say I may never live alone cause each and every day has to be planned out for me and explained to me step-by-step. But I plan to prove everyone wrong.

I plan to show everyone that I am not defined by my disabilities. I am not defined by my Autism.

I plan to show them all that I am a child unlike any other. I intend to show everyone that just because I may be made different that does not mean that I will automatically fall into the same category as all other kids who have the same mental disabilities as me. I am different, and whether people except it or not every child is made differently.

No two Autistic kids are the same. We each have our own journeys and battles that we have to face. We each have our own way of doing things. None of us do things the exact same way. Each of us have our own personalities.

I didn't learn to talk or walk at the same age as most of my peers, but I did learn. Some kids with Autism never learn. Each Autistic child is different and whether the world wants to see and except that or not there is really no two that are exactly alike.

Part two:

The Mothers' View

Chapter 7

I am the mother of an 11-year-old boy named Ricky. I have raised this child for the most part on my own for the most of his life. It has not been a particularly easy journey. There have been many hardships throughout the years.

Especially since he is not my only child, nor is he a particularly easy child to deal with at any given time. However, that is not to say that he is an extremely difficult child either. Yes, Ricky is different than most kids in numerous ways, but he is also the same in many ways.

Ricky started out in life hating it when people held him. He was never an overall very affectionate child, nor does he like it when others are really affectionate with him. He was never a child who would give a lot of hugs or kisses. Though he was one who loved it when you talked to him or sang to him.

Let's go into the history a little bit... my son was born on a cold morning in December. No one was in the delivery room with me when I had him. His father never even knew he was born until many years later. Though that was not because of me.

You see Ricky's dad walked away when I was 5 months pregnant and never looked back. That was not good, but it did not hurt how I raised my son. There have been times when I have doubted whether I could handle taking care of him and his sisters on my own.

However, I managed to do just that for almost 9 years. Than I met my husband, and now we raise the kids together, but I am jumping ahead of myself. I am going to begin from the beginning and go forward. That will be the easiest way to document Ricky and who he is to me.

Ricky is an extraordinary child and he has for the most part always been a somewhat different child. You see unlike my girls, Ricky did not talk at a very early age. Instead he stayed silent until he was five years old. Then even though he was talking he was not talking a lot or very clearly.

His words came in spurts and short verses. At times he would say things that were clear and easy to identify and yet at other times the words that came out of him were impossible to understand. However, his older sister always seemed to know exactly what he was saying.

You see whereas my oldest was an extremely gifted little girl for her age, my boy always seemed to lag just a little behind on the milestones that I already seen her surpass. I never really thought much about it though until he was years old and not walking or talking. That is when I began to worry that something was wrong.

So, I took him into the doctor and asked them why he was not walking or talking, and they ran a bunch of tests and came back with the first result that would shake up my world. I mean being a for all intents and purposes single mother it was going to be difficult to handle three kids and numerous adjustments for my son.

They came back and told me that his first unofficial diagnosis was Pervasive Developmental Disorder-not otherwise specifies, otherwise known as PDD-NOS. With that diagnosis came also the suggestion that we call and get him set up with Babies Can't Wait, so that they could send a therapist out to the house to help him. We were able to get that set up and they sent out a therapist to teach him ASL (American Sign Language), so that he would be able to communicate with the rest of us.

They also taught him his major body parts and taught us the same signs so that we could communicate. They continued to come out to the house and work with him until almost his third birthday. After his third birthday they decided to move him over to the special needs school out of Thomaston. That is when life became even more exciting.

Chapter 8

The first year of him being in school was pretty easy. He loved his bus driver. She was so sweet and kind with him. She would pick him up right at the house in our front yard which made things super easy for us.

He started taking speech classes and begin learning how to talk and say even more. He even began to walk better, though it was mostly on his tiptoes. It was during his second year in the special needs school that he discovered his voice and actually began to put together understandable words and sentences. Then life really got interesting.

During his second year he got into his first bit of trouble, by throwing things and showing out. Nothing super major though. They were able to handle the problem at school and then told me about it later.

He stayed at the special needs school until he reached five years old then we moved him to regular school when he started pre-kindergarten. His pre-kindergarten year was pretty uneventful. He didn't have any major problems that year.

I don't remember much from his kindergarten year. The next year was his first-grade year.

That was the first year he really got into some major trouble. He had gotten into trouble for throwing things and the teacher had to call the principal to the room to get him. However, instead of toting him directly to his office the principal only toted him out of the classroom. When he sat my son down outside the room, Ricky reared back and kicked him.

After he did that, he took off back into the room and hid under a desk. He refused to come out. The school ended up having to call me to come to the school and get him out from under the desk. I followed the techniques that had been taught to me when all of this first started. I went to the school and they took me back to the classroom where he was at.

I sat down on the floor and talked to him and coaxed him out from under the table where he was hiding. As I spoke to him, he crawled out and sat down in my lap. With that being done I stood him up on the floor and stood up myself, then we walked to the principal's office and talked to him. The principal recommended a paddling, but I had never allowed that at school for my daughter and really was not thrilled with the idea of it being done to my son. Though in the end I did allow him to be paddled. Not that it helped anything, because in the end my son just looked at the principal and told him it didn't hurt him.

Chapter 9

The following year we moved to Forsyth and the kids started school over there. That is when he started second grade, and it was the first year that him and both of his sisters were in the same school. This was the second year that he had gotten into real trouble. It was also the first time that he got hurt.

That year I received a phone call about him trying to steal Lego blocks from his teacher's classroom. I was not happy to say the least. I was even less happy when I was told that another student had pulled my son off the jungle gym at school. I ended up having to take him to the hospital and have his arm x-rayed. There we were told that he had sprained his arm and would be in a sling for a week.

That did not stop him from going to school though. He continued to get up and go. All of his friends were big helps as was his teacher. They all worked with him while he was hurt to help him get what he needed done. They all signed his sling and made him feel good about himself.

During the kids' summer break, I had met the man who that fall became my husband and we went to Virginia to see my family and ended up staying. The kids were put into school there and Ricky started his third-grade year. He hardly ever got into trouble that year. He had a few times that he was spoken to about talking a lot, but there was no major trouble with him.

That fall I married my husband, and he became the kids step-dad and even though he is strict with them the kids adore him. Sometimes he seems stricter with Ricky, but I guess that is a good thing. Hopefully that will help Ricky turn out the way that he is supposed to and become the man that he is meant to be when he grows up.

Chapter 10

We moved back to Georgia the following summer and moved back into our house that we had here. The kids went back to their school where their friends were, and Ricky started his Fourth-grade year. The beginning of the year was easy, and he didn't get into much trouble. It was near the end of the school year that the trouble began.

He joined the band his fourth-grade year and the Lego League otherwise known as Robotics. He tested into the band with the highest score in his school. I was so proud of him. He also was enthralled with the idea of being able to build and control robots. I thought the year was going to be a good one with no trouble. However, I thought wrong as I would soon find out.

Near the end of the year I got the call that he had been caught stealing a book from the book fair. This upset me, and I ended up using the same thing that the cop had done with him when he got caught stealing from the stores. I made him sit down and write a letter of apology to his principal, his teacher, and his librarian. Then the next day I drove him to school.

I went with him to hand his letter to his principal and she explained to me that he was going to have to spend a half day in ISS (In School Suspension). I totally agreed with her. Then I went with him to give his letter to his teacher and the librarian, but we only were able to find his teacher. So, the principal said she would make sure he took the other letter to the librarian later in the day. The rest of the year was uneventful, and I was thankful of that.

Chapter 11

This past year was his fifth-grade year and it was pretty well uneventful. He was still in band but decided to drop it a couple weeks into the school year. We were in Forsyth until Christmas break and then we moved to South Georgia closer to my dad and his side of the family. Closer to the beach, which we all love to visit whenever we can get to it. Which unfortunately has not been a whole lot this past year.

With the move Ricky decided to rejoin the band at his new school. The year remained uneventful throughout the rest of the school year. He graduated fifth grade and moved onto the middle school. I am proud of the young man he is becoming and the man he will be when he is grown.

This year he is a sixth-grader, he is still in the band. This year he even tried out for and made the football team. Though he quit after the first game, because he did not agree with having a coach that cussed at the team. This year he got his second ISS for hitting another little boy who had been on the football team with him.

Then just before Thanksgiving break and our move to my grandmothers he got his next ISS for farting during an active shooter lockdown at his school. Which was a bit of a shock to me, but I could understand why it was a big deal. During the kids Thanksgiving break we made the move over to my grandmothers. Now we live with her and help her however necessary.

When I first found out about what the doctor's thought was wrong with Ricky I was in shock. I did not want to believe that there was anything wrong with him. Sometimes I still do not believe it. I honestly believe that he is what controls his actions and the things that he does. Yes, the doctors may say that he is Autistic, but his Autism is not what defines him as a person.

Chapter 12

My first impression of my son when the doctors told me his diagnosis was that they were lying. All I could think was that there was no way that it was true. That he was not what they said he was nor was his diagnosis what controlled his actions or reactions. I honestly thought that the doctor was pulling my chain, and they were just using a really big medical term to tell me that my child was a trouble maker.

When Ricky was little, I knew that there was something going on with him. He was not developing the way that a normal child should have been developing. Though I never expected the diagnosis that he received when I took him in to see the doctor.

Ricky is an overall intelligent little boy. He loves anything with wheels on it. He holds a huge interest in video games as well. He is a very hyper little boy and at times I think he could stand to slow down just a bit.

As I have been told by his doctors it is Autism Spectrum Disorder, ADHD, and ODD. Though I will be completely honest and say that I do not believe that those are what define him. He is not the medical terms that they have used for him. He may have those disorders, but they are not what makes up the boy that he is at all.

His school grades are amazing for having faced the challenges that he has in his 11 years. He is an A and B student. His behavior at school could be better, but he is not a tremendous troublemaker. That's not to say that he has not been in trouble at school.

I do not know if I believe what the doctors say at all. I do know that there was something wrong with him to keep him from developing when he should have or like he should have when he was younger. However, I do not believe that the diagnosis's that the doctors have pinned on him are what has been the root of his problems at all.

I do not believe that, because contrary to what some may think Ricky can understand right from wrong. He may not always understand that something he has done is wrong at the moment that he does it, but he does understand the difference.

Ricky is an extremely talented little boy in somethings. He just sometimes allows his attitude and anger to get the best of him, and when it does, he cannot always control his actions or reactions to things.

The Autism is not what defines nor is it what controls him. He controls himself and decides on his own what he is doing at any given moment. Now that is not to say that this is what is true for all kids with this disability, but mine has more control over his actions than he would like people to think that he does.

Part Three:
The Father's View

Chapter 13

When I first met Ricky, he was 8 years old. My first impression of him was that he was an overly hyper little boy. He was constantly causing his mama problems and getting on her nerves. It was obvious that he had not had a stable male father figure in his life ever.

I started trying to be of help to her early on, but I wasn't sure how far to take the discipline with him without upsetting her. Though she never really said much to me when I did get on to him or his sisters. I have enjoyed having them all in my life. The kids are good for the most part.

However, when I was first told what he was diagnosed with I did not believe it and still do not believe it. I actually just believe that he needs a strong male figure in his life. Someone who will be willing to bust his tail when he needs it and not back down from him.

If I had to describe Ricky, oI would say that he is an extremely hyper little boy. He could bare to learn when he needs to sit down and chill out and not get on people's nerves. I would also say that he should have had his butt busted a lot more often when he was younger. If that had happened, he may not have turned out as wild as he is today.

I was told his official diagnosis is ASD, ADHD, and ODD. That maybe what the doctors are saying, but I believe that what he really needed was a strong, and stable man in his life with a firm hand for the start. Though I could be wrong and that may not have helped at all, but I believe that it would have.

His school work is amazing. He is a A and B student in school. He participates in the band and has participated in the Lego League as well. He has even playing football for the school, but he did not like. He can be a little troublemaker at school, but he is not a huge problem in school. He has just caused some problems at times.

His likes are the same as most normal boys. However, his big dislike is having to listen to anyone. He does not like being told what to do or how to do anything. He has a strong dislike for anyone who gets on to him or tells him how to do things.

I do not believe the diagnosis that the doctor told his mother. Yes, they may be correct, but I believe that it is more him needing a strong hand to discipline him than anything else. Without a strong male figure with a strong hand for discipline then he could grow up to be a real trouble maker type and land somewhere that he really doesn't need to be at all.

Chapter 14

I know that this child is not a true trouble maker and I hope that with my guidance I can help him to make something out of himself. That way instead of him messing up and ending up in a jail or prison somewhere instead he will be successful and make something out of himself. This boy is all time telling me that he wants to be in the Air Force and I hope that I can help to guide him onto that path.

My sincerest hope for him is that he becomes all that he can be and really makes some thing of himself. I know that anything less than accomplishing his potential would hurt his mother deeply. I hope with my strong hand and know how of different things I can help him to become a man that people will admire and look up too.

A man of honor and trust rather than one that lies and deceives. Someone that his mother, his sisters and I can all be proud of to call their family. These are my hopes for him as a person and as a man. I hope that he can see that I do not get on to him just to be disciplining him, but rather I get on to him to help him learn what is right and wrong.

Part Four:
The Sisters' View

Chapter 15

Hi my name is Lillian and I have known my brother since he was born and my mother brought him home from the hospital. My mom says my first thoughts about my baby brother was "when can we take him back mom." I guess I had gotten used to being an only child, I was three months from being 2 years old when he was born.

However, as I got older and watched my brother grow, I gained a new impression of him. Now my impression of him is to question why he is out of control and such a brat? He is constantly getting on my nerves or our moms' nerves.

He is constantly wanting to show out or fight with my and our younger sister. I try really hard to get along with him, but sometimes it is just so hard that I get frustrated with him. Than once I get frustrated, I no longer want to play with him anymore.

The only thing I think is wrong with my brother is that he has anger issues. Also, he can never own up to anything that he has done that is wrong. He would rather lie to our mom than actually take responsibility for the thing that he may have done that was wrong. I have gotten into trouble many times because of him.

Though there have also been a few times that I have taken the blame for him. I do it because I do not seeing my brother or sister get into trouble. It makes me sad when they get into trouble or when one of us gets in trouble because of one of the others.

Chapter 16

My opinion of my brother is that he is bossy, annoying, and mouthy. He loves bossing me and our sister around. He also likes being annoying when it comes to our sister and I all the time. He is always telling us what to do and how to do it. Not to mention he is all the time being mouthy with the grownups, rather to our mom or our stepdad.

His biggest issue far as I can tell is his anger. He is all the time getting angry over the littlest things. I do not understand how he can get so upset over the littlest things. It doesn't matter what is going on if he doesn't like it, he will get angry.

Now at school he does pretty good to the best of my knowledge. He is a little out of control at times on the bus, but not a lot. He is always super talkative on the bus. I would also think that he is talkative in his classes to, though I hope that he isn't as bad as he is on the bus.

He likes cars and anything else that has wheels on it. He also likes soccer and playing video games. He is fascinated with racing and race cars too. He hates being bored, knowing that he is not the boss or being told what to do at any time. He also hates being told No for anything.

I do not believe what the doctors say about my brother. I think that my brother is just a brat and a true pain in the butt. Sometimes he gets on my nerves so much, but at times he is also fun to have around. He is fun when he wants to be, and he comes up with some fun games to play to at times.

I love my brother don't get me wrong, but sometimes he gets on my nerves so much. Sometimes I would like to trade him in, but other times I wouldn't trade him for anything in the world. I enjoy playing different games with him and spending time with him. I hope my moms' book about my brother will help others to understand that Autism is not always bad. I also hope that her book helps to give others hope for the future.

Chapter 17

Hi, my name is Star, and this is my thoughts on my older brother. I am the baby and both of my siblings are older than me. Hopefully what I say here will help others to understand what it is like having an older brother who has Autism.

My first impression of my brother was that he was crazy and annoying. He sometimes gets on our older sisters' nerves. I do not know if he means to do it, but he is always doing something that bothers her. He sometimes gets on my nerves to, but now as much as he gets on our sister Lillian's nerves.

He even gets on our moms and dad's nerves sometimes. Whether or not he does it on purpose to irritate them, but he does get on their nerves. I do not really understand my brother, but I like being able to play with him when he is not being annoying. His games are super fun at times.

He is not good at helping people with things when he does not want to in the house or on the outside of the house. He can also be very rude, and he is horrible at making and keeping commitments. I also think that he needs to stop talking so much.

Sometimes he talks more than he should and that to gets on everyone's nerves.

He is good in school grade wise, but he gets angry at the teachers and other students really easy. When that happens, he usually ends up in the principal's office or ISS. He sometimes finds it easy to make friends and sometimes hard. He likes playing all kinds of games, especially if there are cars involved in the game.

He does not like playing barbies, stuffed animal games or horse games with me and our sister. That makes us sad sometimes, because we wish he would play with us. I suppose in my opinion as his little sister some of what the doctors say maybe true, but I really do not know. I honestly believe that there has to be something making him so hyper and angry all the time.

I don't know if what I have shared will help others to understand my brother or not, but I do hope that it will help others to understand that all children with Autism are not the same. I have Autism myself, but I was not behind on any of my development other than my speech. I talk when I want to and to who I want to and if I don't want to talk than I just stay quiet.

The Conclusion

Chapter 18

With the telling of this book I hope to help others who have a loved one, sibling, or child living with Autism. By telling this story and giving the opinions of each of Ricky's family members I hope to help show that Autism doesn't just affect the person that has that diagnosis. Instead it affects all connected to that person.

Autism is not just suffered by the one who has the diagnosis, but it is instead felt by all connected to them. By telling the story from the side of each of his family members and offering their thoughts I hope it helps. Autism is not a disease that is contagious like the flu, the common cold, or pneumonia, but it is something that every person who loves the one who has it will feel.

Being a child with Autism is difficult as I have seen through my son. However, being a parent or sibling of a child with Autism is also difficult. Most especially when you never know what that child's attitude or mindset will be like when they wake up in the morning. I have raised two children with Autism, one is soon to be 12 years old and the other is 11 years old, and each of them are as different as night and day.

You would never know by looking at them that their brains are wired completely different from yours or mine. Without knowing their back stories, their successes and their downfalls you would never guess that they have their issues mentally. They act as normal as they possibly can when they can, but they have their little offsets that set them apart from other children their own age.

I hope that my journey and my sons' journey can help others to understand that Autism is not something to be feared. It is not something to look down on a person for, or something to pick on a person about, it is just who that person is, and it will not change.

www.ingramcontent.com/pod-product-compliance
Lightning Source LLC
Chambersburg PA
CBHW051420250726
48655CB00003B/1143